The Road To

Romance

Getting To The Heart Of Love

And Connection

Mary Franklin .C.

Mary Franklin.C.

Copyright@2023Mary Franklin .C.

Table Of Content

Mary Franklin.C.

Introduction

Imagine being in a partnership that is brimming with romance, caring, companionship, respect, and a complete feeling of duty. a remarkable union marked by contentment, amusement, delight, and unfathomable kinship.

You may construct and grow the exceptional and unique sort of connection you've been longing for with the help of this educational book. From wherever you are right now in your romantic life, it is a trip that will lead you to

a new location filled with immense satisfaction and joy.

You must be aware that the process is the same despite

the kind of connection you hope to have with the person

you love. A friendship is not a situation that starts to

blossom right away since everything in life has periods

of ups and downs, so to build a really solid, enduring

connection, it's necessary to put forth patience,

diligence, and devotion.

The benefits are certain and well worthwhile. Furthermore, this book will teach you what it takes to manage and handle the obstacles, challenges, and benefits of having an enjoyable partnership.

You must realize, as a lover, that romantic partnerships are more difficult than we often imagine. You may build an affair that is incredibly loving, attentive, supportive, and fulfilling with the right steps.

Well, inside this book, you can pick up the abilities and knowledge required to create a connection that can remarkably withstand the test of time.

Before you can be an outstanding spouse to the one you love, you have to develop a love for oneself and build what is known as self-love. You will discover how to form wholesome routines and constructive thought patterns that will promote your well-being and significantly enhance your relationship.

The Road To Romance

Any partnership that wants to be healthy has to have

clear limits.

Boundaries ensure that it's a possibility for you and the

person you love to feel respected and heard while also

fostering a sense of safety and security.

Working on your mental agility, or the capacity to

comprehend and manage both your own and your

lover's feelings is necessary if you want to be in a good

relationship. It is one of the nicest aspects of creating a

strong bond with your spouse and growing into their ideal match.

So, if you want to be a good partner and build a connection that is based on love and affection, you must appreciate the value of the trip. This book will take you on a personal growth and self-discovery trip to get you ready for starting a last friendship with the one you love.

Chapter One

Turning Your Engine For A Romance

You have to be absolutely certain your engine is fired up and prepared to go before starting towards the road to romance. This chapter will greatly assist you in igniting your engine so that you can head out on your adventure with enthusiasm and assurance.

Self-Love

You must cultivate what we refer to as self-love to have

a good friendship. It will be very difficult for you to love

and connect with those around you if you don't love

yourself first.

You can gain the ability to cherish and

appreciate yourself, and once you do that, you are going

to be willing to generously and genuinely experience

love from others. Once you do this, then would be willing to extend that unconditional affection to others.

The physical, mental, and emotional aspects of self-love are its three essential elements. Exercising serves as one of its core elements when it comes to love for oneself. Our state of mind and emotions are greatly influenced by exercise in addition to our physical wellness. It supports a happier mood, increased self-esteem, and stress reduction.

Keeping Your Oil Fresh With Honesty

One crucial concept you must grasp is that honesty is like the oil that supports a friendship flowing and operating smoothly. It serves as a kind of lube that keeps the conversations in your friendship flowing and eliminates all friction.

If you fail to establish a connection with one another (your lover), it's simple to go into disagreements with the someone you love. Being truthful and forthright about how you feel and ideas is a tried and true method

of building connections.

Even though it may be difficult and troubling, you must

be completely honest about how you perceive things

and the things you think. It furthermore has to do with

speaking what's real rather than keeping it a secret

within you; even if you worry that your lover may not

concur with all that you are suggesting or be pleased

about it, you shouldn't let that stop you from speaking

your mind.

Staying right about your behavior is a crucial aspect of honesty. This has to do with refusing to act dishonestly or withholding details from someone you love.

Being willing to identify your errors and acknowledge the blame for them is another aspect of being truthful. Creating a strong connection built on transparency and confidence requires you to accept your mistake.

Being a good partner calls for being forthright and frank about one's requirements, desires, and boundaries. An additional aspect of honesty you shouldn't joke with is the need to be completely forthcoming about what you're interested in your partnership with the person you love and what you are not ready to make sacrifices on.

As a lover, you have to figure out how to be sincere and forthright with your partner, and listening intently is a vital component of a loving relationship. The ability to listen to your spouse and make an effort to grasp their point of view is known as active listening. It entails being receptive to hearing words that you would not normally love to hear.

It is very important to address a dispute or argument you are having with your spouse with empathy and compassion. It has to do with considering your partner's viewpoint and being prepared to make concessions.

In order to resolve a problem or disagreement with your spouse, you must first put your attention on the situation at hand rather than on the other person.

You should concentrate all of your efforts on resolving the issue rather than criticizing or assaulting your lover.

Separating your partner from the problem is essential, despite the fact that it might be quite difficult. Using the "I" phrase is another smart tactic for resolving disputes. Instead of expressing, "You never listen to me," when you are having a disagreement with your spouse, you may say, "I feel like my needs aren't being heard." I hope you can understand how important the "I" statement is while trying to work out a disagreement with your spouse.

Taking a pause if the discussion becomes too tense. You and your spouse will have some time to cool down and collect your thoughts after this.

Keeping Your Coolant Cool With Empathy

Understanding your partner's viewpoint and placing yourself in their position are the only requirements for empathy. It is vital to consider things from your partner's perspective rather than putting a lot of emphasis on your own.

The Road To Romance

Well, having empathy may be quite difficult, especially

when you're extremely irate, irritated, or annoyed. But

you must always remember to give it a go. You should

attempt to resolve the issue since a loving spouse

wouldn't point the finger or place blame on their

partner.

Another cool approach to be cool with empathy is to

have a cheerful attitude. In spite of having a difficult

talk, it involves highlighting the positive aspects of your

friendship.

You may do this by being able to say nice things about your partner even while you are engaged in a disagreement.

Although it is really significant, it is not that simple to deal with. The more optimistic you are when having a challenging talk, the simpler it will be to work out the differences with the person you love.

You must refrain from being defensive. This has to do with not becoming angry or defensive when your spouse vents their frustrations or worries. But you must completely concentrate on comprehending their

viewpoint.

Mary Franklin.C.

Chapter Two

Driving On The Road To Romance

Potholes Of Jealousy

Accepting that jealousy is a common experience despite

the fact it is obviously harmful is important. When it's

out of control or excessive, jealousy poses a serious

threat to a partnership. Destructive actions may result

from it.

There are a few techniques to manage envy in a healthy way. Identifying the root causes of your envy is the first step. It is very important to find and resolve the fundamental cause of insecurity since jealousy frequently has this as its foundation.

The next step is to talk to your spouse about your sentiments in a cordial, composed, and polite manner, once you have identified and addressed the source of your envy.

The Road To Romance

You ought to stay away from creating unneeded

controversy, leveling accusations, or assigning blame. On

the contrary, you ought to concentrate entirely on how

you are feeling at the moment and what your lover

needs from you.

Another great approach for controlling jealousy is

staying focused on the good parts of your romantic

partnership. When you suffer from jealousy, it tends to

be simple to fall victim to bad ideas and emotions, but it

is very helpful to keep in mind all the positive aspects

of the connection you have.

Mary Franklin.C.

An additional crucial method for minimizing jealous

conduct within your romantic connection is to practice

taking care of yourself. One certain strategy to help

yourself reduce feelings of jealousy and insecurity is to

take good care of your physical and emotional needs.

Having a nutritious diet, getting adequate rest, and

doing things that make you happy and joyful are all vital

components of self-care. The act of envy can also be

reduced by concentrating on your objective and area of

interest.

The Road To Romance

You're less likely to feel threatened by your partner's

success or accomplishment when you're fully committed

to your objective. Building your self-esteem via it is a

fantastic idea.

Allowing life's activity to take over is a lovely approach

to lessen the act of jealousy, but it's crucial to make time

for your spouse while you're together.

This entails scheduling a date night or making time for a

meaningful talk. You must engender trust in your

partnership. In order to overcome the act of envy, trust

is crucial. Honesty, respect, and keeping your word are a

few amazing methods to develop trust with your spouse.

Signpost of Support

Being available to someone you care about whenever

they're in need of you and supporting their feelings are

examples of supportive acts. Observe carefully.

Unquestionably, listening to others without making a

decision and giving them your whole attention is a good

thing to do. At all costs, you must put this crucial part

of your relationship into action.

Another crucial form of assistance that you could use to strengthen your bond with your spouse is to support both personally and professionally. Becoming your couple's biggest fan is the most crucial component of assistance.

It is crucial to wish your spouse luck in his endeavors. A further fantastic way to assist is to communicate safety and surveillance.

The latter has something to do with helping the person you love throughout times of difficulty and providing a shoulder to weep on is an advantageous way to show

support.

A tried-and-true way of offering support is to say thanks.

Making the person you love feel valuable and

illustrating how thankful you are for their love can go a

long way toward making you a nice lover.

Being supportive could assist you and the person you

love to become more connected and understanding of

one another. It contributes to a relationship's sense of

safety and comfort. You feel safer and more

comfortable when you know you can rely on the one

you love.

How do you show support to one you love through a

difficult time? Listen carefully; it's not always necessary

to provide advice or solutions when your spouse simply

needs to talk.

Assure and inspire. Inform your spouse of your

wholehearted trust in them and that you believe that

they are capable of handling any issues they are now

facing. For instance, if your spouse is struggling with a

work project, offer to brainstorm with them or

proofread their writing.

Chapter Three

Adventures On The Road To Romance

Sidetracked By Insecurity And Detours Of Self-doubt

One of the main ways that insecurity can cause detours on the path to love is through anxiety over one's incapacity. Imagine Diana, for instance, being able to display her artwork at a gallery but feeling anxious about the criticism and the artwork's lack of quality.

As a consequence of this issue, the artist decides not to take advantage of the chance to share their art with the entire world. The fear of failure may prevent people from acting appropriately.

Angst over potential risks is another form of instability that can result in a lack of self-confidence. Imagine Diana is shy and uncomfortable speaking to others because she worries about being judged or deemed unimportant.

The Road To Romance

She ultimately keeps her sentiments to herself and doesn't have any meaningful interactions with other people. While managing this dread and uncertainty may be difficult, it's important to remember that they do not have the power to control our actions.

It is really easy to get beyond this difficulty and develop a solid bond with your partner if you put in a little work and practice. Being able to communicate honestly and freely with the person you love is an excellent method to get over your fear.

We must properly discuss our wants, ideas, and emotions with our partners. This will assist in the relationship's growth of confidence and empathy. A partner must understand the value of honest exchanges to keep their connection strong.

Setting limits that are reasonable is a great additional tactic. This implies that you must communicate your needs and wants to your companion. You can set a restriction and let your lover know about it, for example, if you don't want him or her to use each others phone.

The Road To Romance

We will now see how to implement these tactics in specific scenarios. Imagine that you are upset because your lover is spending time with someone else. How can I use these suggestions in this circumstance?

Respect your dissatisfaction at first. Be sure you understand the powerful emotion that is underneath jealousy. One may feel pressured or uneasy.

If you are aware of how you are feeling, you may attempt attempt to control the situation by utilizing open communication and compassion. Even though it may require some work and time, this technique can be a powerful tool for creating long-lasting connections.

This strategy may also be applied in this manner. Consider that you both have anxiety and a desire to relax. You may show that you are present and eager to listen by following the tips below. Take away your phone and give your lover your whole attention.

You may also convey your attention and engagement by using your body language. As soon as possible, check to see whether your sentiments are true and if it's okay

for you to feel this way.

Chapter Four

Pit stops Along The Way

Gas Stations Of Gratitude

A powerful feeling like gratefulness has the power to alter a relationship. One of the most effective ways to express gratitude is to pay attention to and value the little things. For instance, your partner could value the preparation of the meals, the purchase of your preferred beverage each time they go shopping, or the disposal of the trash.

We acknowledge and express our gratitude for these little objects as we replenish the symbolic gas tank. When you're in a dilemma, it could be challenging to think of basic things. Making a list of your evaluations, no matter how significant or insignificant, is a useful activity.

Rest Area Of Understanding

Having a healthy affair with the one we love requires understanding, we must continue to listen to our spouse. To do this, we need to change our strategy and put more effort into comprehending your viewpoint. It might be quite challenging to regulate our emotions when we are angry or upset, but we must try.

Understanding is important since it improves our relationship. If our partner feels heard and understood, they are more willing to open up to us and express their feelings. Making space for intimacy and vulnerability also requires that we share our ideas and feelings with others.

Another outstanding skill regarding the balance of understanding is having the capacity to relate to another person's feelings, which is a form of empathy. Sympathy, or the state of feeling distressed for a person, varies from empathy.

Empathy enables us to see things from our partner's viewpoint and put ourselves in their position. The use of "I message" is one method we might develop empathy. Here, we may convey our feelings without making numerical references to our companion.

For instance, we may say, "I get irritated when I see the dishes in the sink," as opposed to, "You always leave your dishes in the sink.

Chapter Five

Roadside Attractions Of Affection

Stop And Smell The Rose Of Appreciation

When we take a moment to cherish what our lover does for us. We are actually letting them know that we are grateful even for the little gestures and that we cherish them. When your spouse does anything for you uttering the word thank you is usually not okay you also need to be able to acknowledge and value them

Take A Selfie At The Landmark Of Laughter

All of this is done to make sure that both of you

are happy. Finding ways to have fun with the one you

love in this scenario is crucial. It is so straightforward to

attempt to make them feel emotional or to tell a good

story about the partnership.

You might also play video games with each other to

make them feel loved. Participating in things or activities

that your partner enjoys or finds enjoyable is an

excellent opportunity to connect, laugh, and have fun

together.

You may also influence others to speak in jest by watching a fun movie or walking in the park. It's crucial to identify things that would make you both happy and strengthen your relationship.

Finding things that both of you like and that strengthen your relationship is the key. To be considered admiration or laughing, an activity need not be large or complicated.

The tiniest moment may occasionally have the largest influence. For instance, sending a humorous text message to your spouse, writing a love note for them, or

simply grinning and laughing with them while you're

talking. It's also vital to note that humor and expressions

of gratitude aren't necessarily crucial in a love

partnership. They play a significant role in interpersonal,

familial, and professional connections as well.

Chapter Six

Weather Along The Way

Stormy Skies Of Conflict

Conflict may be a regular and beneficial component of

every bond, much like a stormy sky. What counts is how

we respond to it. Do you believe that it is possible to

handle conflict healthily and politely when it is raging?

I'd want for you to know that the essential strategy for

navigating the turbulent skies of conflict is

communication. Even when we are angry, being able to express our needs and feel respected can enable us to overcome disagreement.

It's also crucial to be open to hearing what the other person has to say and comprehending their viewpoints. You must take a break when tensions between you and your partner rise. This will enable you to feel more at ease and come up with solutions.

Sunny Days Of Love

How can we make sure that there is a lot of love

between us? A small act of appreciation and compassion

may make a big difference. Whether it's a hug, a nice

remark, or a considerate action, this lovely moment may

make your partner's day.

That brief time frame has the power to lay a solid

foundation of love and trust. Similar to a garden,

relationships require attention and maintenance; the

more effort we put into them, the more we will get from

them.

Mary Franklin.C.

It's crucial to enjoy yourself in a relationship. Being a good partner also requires you to work well with others as a team.

Chapter Seven

A Map Of The Future

Points Of Interest

The points of interest can include everything we anticipate, including weddings, trips, birthdays, and a host of other events. We need to develop as a couple and learn from each other. Supporting one another is crucial for further growth. This could have to do with supporting one another as we work toward our objectives and discover new passions.

Additionally, sharing memories fosters closeness and connection. A lasting impression may be made on a relationship by sharing memories with your loved ones. Even in the near future, your spouse could recall the sensation of sharing a beach sunset with you or the aroma of your favorite food.

Uncharted Territory

uncharted territory can be scary but it is as well a very vital part of a partnership which makes it to be a little more exciting. It can be as simple as trying out a new restaurant, or as big as moving to a new city. it's crucial in opening up a new experience and new problem with your lover. A willingness to take risks and try new things together can make one's partnership more dynamic, and fulfilling it can also help you and your partner to grow as a partner.

Mary Franklin.C.

Chapter Eight

The Destination Of Happiness

Do you believe that happiness is something you can experience once and then hang onto, or do you believe it to be more of a journey that you continually traveling toward? Like getting married, purchasing a new house or vehicle, or other one-time goals, finding happiness may also be a life long journey.

The road is consistent, even though the goal may change. If you simply saw pleasure as a goal, it would be quite simple to become disheartened. However, there are more possibilities to discover happiness in each moment if you consistently place emphasis on what you appreciate.

Do you believe that concentrating solely on the trip rather than the objective carries any risk? Yes! If you're simply thinking about the route, you run the risk of getting complacent. It's similar to going on a trek and losing focus on the route because you're enjoying the landscape so much.

So keeping an eye on the goal achieves the ideal balance. Flexibility is a further aspect of the balance. You risk losing patience if you go lost or experience an unexpected event if you are too intent on getting to your objective.

However, if you are concentrating on the road, you risk losing sight of your goal. Therefore, the trick is to be adaptable enough to alter directions as required, while simultaneously attempting to maintain focus on the eventual result.

The Joy Of Love

Joy may be described as a slight sense of lightness in the heart as if there were a tiny joyful radiance emanating from inside. It may also be a sense of fulfillment and happiness, as though everything is going just according to plan.

And occasionally, joy might be accompanied by an exhilarating sensation of being on top of the world. Love may evoke feelings of intense kinship and connection to someone or something. It can also give you a strong sense of comfort and safety as if someone would always be there to help you.

And occasionally, falling in love can cause an intense emotional rush that makes you feel as though you could pass out.

Mary Franklin.C.

Chapter Nine

The Journey Never Ends, The Adventure Continues

In the end, the tale of our life never completely ends, no matter how many travels we make back or undertake in our partnership. There is always more to discover in terms of knowledge, experiences, and enjoyment.

So let's continue on our journey with an open mind, keep going, and have fun! The quest to satisfaction in

Mary Franklin.C.

our relationship never ends, to put it simply. The journey

and the goal are both important.

Chapter Ten

Conclusion

The Road To Romance guides you on an adventure of self-discovery, relationship, and love and teaches you how to be a wonderful companion. We set out on this adventure in search of connection and love. We learned what it takes to maintain genuine pleasure in our union.

Along the road, we discover the benefits of being honest, of being aware of who we are and what we want in a relationship. We learned the importance of love, empathy, and transparency in fostering our bond. We were able to see that connection is something we actively nurture in our relationship rather than something that just happens to us.

Along the way, we learned the value of communicating our emotions to our partners and listening to them with understanding and compassion. The most significant connections are not always the simplest to make, but they are always worthwhile of the work and difficulties, as we were about to learn.

The Road To Romance

Finally, we learned that genuine love is a decision we

make every day to take care of and support the people

we love rather than merely a sensation.